QUESTIONS AND ANSWERS
IN SLEEP APNEA
(AN INTERNIST'S PERSPECTIVE)

QUESTIONS AND ANSWERS IN SLEEP APNEA
IN SLEEP APNEA
(AN INTERNIST'S PERSPECTIVE)

Gautam Soparkar

Copyright © 2009 by Gautam Soparkar.

Library of Congress Control Number:		2009905304
ISBN:	Hardcover	978-1-4415-4129-1
	Softcover	978-1-4415-4128-4

This book was printed in the United States of America.

To order additional copies of this book, contact:
Xlibris Corporation
1-888-795-4274
www.Xlibris.com
Orders@Xlibris.com
61150

CONTENTS

SECTION 2: SLEEP STUDIES AND RELATED
TESTS FOR APNEA

SECTION 3: SLEEP APNEA AND SELECTED MEDICAL CONDITIONS

SECTION 4: SELECTED MANAGEMENT ISSUES

INTRODUCTION

There are many excellent textbooks on sleep disorders, but most of them are directed either toward the practicing sleep medicine professional or someone training to be one. As well, although most referrals to a sleep laboratory are for *sleep apnea*, the related books are generally about *sleep medicine* as a whole. As a result, information about sleep apnea tends to be underrepresented and practical information is not readily available for the healthcare provider who suspects sleep apnea, arranges sleep studies, and finally has to act on the results. The purpose of this book is to fill this gap.

It is increasingly obvious that sleep apnea cannot be diagnosed and treated in isolation. It is known to be associated with several medical conditions that fall within the field of the generalist. For this reason, this book looks at sleep apnea from the perspective of an internist rather than a sleep specialist. The relation of sleep apnea to other medical conditions is included, as is sleep apnea in pregnancy and in the perioperative period.

The clinician is faced with four questions about a patient who may have sleep apnea:

- When should I suspect sleep apnea?
- Should I refer the patient for a sleep study?
- What information can I expect from the sleep laboratory?
- What can I do with the information I receive?

This book attempts to answer these and other related questions. The concise approach will hopefully be useful, informative, and help healthcare providers make optimal use of the sleep laboratory. No attempt has been made to give details of the physiology of apnea or the mechanics of continuous positive airway pressure (CPAP); these can be found in more detailed reference books, a selection of which appears in the bibliography. Information about other sleep disorders has been kept to a minimum and appears only in relation to indications for sleep studies.

The book is divided into four sections: (1) "Sleep Apnea: Definitions and Treatment", (2) "Sleep Studies and Related Tests for Apnea", (3) "Sleep Apnea and Selected Medical Conditions", and (4) "Selected Management Issues". I hope the question-and-answer format will be conducive to easy reading and applying in practice. The questions are arranged in what I felt was a logical order.

I am indebted to my patients, whose management has been extremely rewarding and a phenomenal learning experience. Many of the answers were obtained by "reading around" actual patients. Thanks are also due to my colleagues for their support and advice. Many parts of the book are derived from informal discussions and so-called corridor consultations, the value of which cannot be overestimated. I would also like to acknowledge the support of the staff at the Bluewater Sleep Disorder Clinic, Sarnia, and the Leamington Sleep Clinic, Leamington. I am also grateful to my family for showing unflagging patience and support.

Omissions were inevitable due to the compact size of the book. While every effort has been made to ensure accuracy, some errors may have crept in, for which I am solely responsible. Suggestions and comments are welcome and may be sent to soparkar1@gmail.com.

Gautam Soparkar, MBBS, DTCD, MD, MRCP(UK), FRCPC
Adjunct Professor of Medicine
University of Western Ontario
London, Ontario, Canada

DISCLAIMER

This book is directed at healthcare providers and trainees in the healthcare field. It is not meant to be an exhaustive source of information and should not be used as the sole guide in the management of individual patients.

The information contained in this book is not intended to replace professional healthcare advice. It is also not meant to be used for self-diagnosis or self-treatment.

The author and publisher will not be responsible for any losses, injuries, illnesses, or damages arising, either directly or indirectly, from the use of the information contained in this book.

ABBREVIATIONS

AHI: apnea-hypopnea index, the number of apneas and/or hypopneas per hour of sleep

ASV: adaptive servo-ventilation

BiPAP: bilevel positive airway pressure

BMI: body mass index

CHF: congestive heart failure

COPD: chronic obstructive pulmonary disease

CPAP: continuous positive airway pressure

CSA: central sleep apnea

CSR: Cheyne-Stokes respiration

EEG: electroencephalogram

EKG: electrocardiogram

ENT: ear, nose, and throat

EPR: expiratory pressure relief

LAUP: laser-assisted uvuloplasty

MSLT: multiple sleep latency test

NIPPV: noninvasive positive pressure ventilation

OHS: obesity-hypoventilation syndrome

OSA: obstructive sleep apnea

OSAHS: obstructive sleep apnea-hypopnea syndrome (same as OSAS)

OSAS: obstructive sleep apnea syndrome, includes OSA and UARS

PLMD: periodic limb movement disorder

PSG: polysomnogram/polysomnography, sleep study

RBD: REM-behaviour disorder

RDI: respiratory disturbance index

REM: rapid eye movement

RERA: respiratory effort-related arousal
RLS: restless legs syndrome
SDB: sleep-disordered breathing
UARS: upper airway resistance syndrome
UPPP: uvulopalatopharyngoplasty

SECTION 1

SLEEP APNEA:
DEFINITIONS AND TREATMENT

1. What is sleep apnea?

Sleep apnea is a condition characterized by repeated cessation of breathing during sleep. When the cessation of breathing is complete, it is called apnea; incomplete cessation ("shallow breathing" with significant reduction in airflow) is called hypopnea. By convention, the cessation of breathing (complete or partial) should be at least 10 seconds long to be called apnea or hypopnea. The term "sleep apnea" includes both apneas and hypopneas.

2. What are the types of sleep apnea?

The multiplicity of terms is sometimes confusing, but there are two main types (Figure 1):

- *Obstructive sleep apnea (OSA)*. This is the most common type of sleep apnea (90%) and refers to repeated mechanical obstruction of the upper airway where it is collapsible, i.e., between the posterior part of the nose and the larynx.

- *Central sleep apnea (CSA)*. This is much less common (10%) and refers to failure of brainstem impulses to initiate respiration. Common causes include congestive heart failure (CHF), sedation, or a neurological problem. Cheyne-Stokes respiration (CSR) is a special type of CSA characterized by waxing and waning respiratory amplitude. The collective term CSR-CSA is sometimes used.

"Mixed" sleep apnea is a subset of OSA where the apnea begins as the central type and then becomes obstructive. The initial event is cessation of respiratory effort and upper airway collapse followed by resumption of respiratory effort against the obstructed airway. Treatment is the same as that for OSA.

Upper airway resistance syndrome (UARS) can also be considered a subset of OSA under the broader term obstructive sleep apnea syndrome (OSAS)—see question 7.

Obesity-hypoventilation syndrome (OHS) is a condition in which obesity (usually extreme) coexists with reduced ventilatory drive and carbon dioxide retention. This condition often coexists with OSA when the common factor is obesity—see question 9.

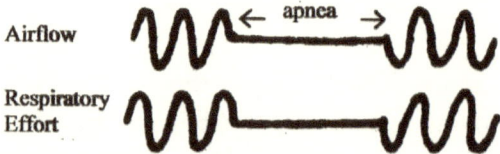

FIGURE 1. OBSTRUCTIVE & CENTRAL APNEA

3. What are the clinical differences between OSA and CSA?

Symptoms of OSA include snoring, witnessed apneas, choking or gasping in sleep, repeated arousals, excessive daytime somnolence, nonrestful sleep, fatigue, and morning headaches. Impotence and symptoms suggesting a mood disorder may also be seen and the condition is sometimes confused with a depressive illness.

In CSA, features of the underlying condition often dominate the clinical picture (e.g., features of CHF, history of narcotic medication, or neurological conditions). CSA is not necessarily associated with snoring since upper airway obstruction is not the problem.

CSA may coexist with OSA, and clinical features of both may be present. Both conditions may be associated with significant daytime symptoms, such as excessive daytime somnolence and fatigue.

The term sleep-disordered breathing (SDB) is often used to include all types of sleep apnea (classical OSA, UARS, OHS, "mixed apnea", and CSA).

4. What does a sleep study (PSG) show in case of OSA and CSA?

With OSA, a PSG would show apneas and/or hypopneas with evidence of respiratory effort, which is intact. The problem is due to repeated mechanical obstruction of the nonrigid part of the upper airway.

With CSA, a PSG would show apneas but with *no* evidence of respiratory effort since the problem is that of initiation of respiration rather than mechanical obstruction.

5. What is the apnea-hypopnea index (AHI), and how is it useful?

The apnea-hypopnea index (AHI) is the average number of apneas and/or hypopneas per hour of sleep, i.e., (apneas + hypopneas) / sleep time in hours = AHI.

The AHI is used to determine the severity of sleep apnea. By convention, the following classification of severity is used for adults:

AHI <5 = normal
AHI 5-15 = mild apnea
AHI 15-30 = moderate apnea
AHI >30 = severe apnea

This is an oversimplification and the classification is not perfect since severity depends not only on the number of apneas and hypopneas but also on other factors such as number of arousals and oxygen desaturation. Still, this classification is commonly used in interpreting PSGs.

6. What is the respiratory disturbance index (RDI)?

This is a newer term that includes not only apneas and hypopneas but also other events which indicate sleep disturbance due to respiratory events, including so-called respiratory effort-related arousals (RERAs). All such events per hour is termed the respiratory disturbance index (RDI).

The RDI has often been used interchangeably with the AHI although, strictly speaking, they are not the same. The RDI may eventually replace the AHI in common usage, but the AHI has been used in this book because of its simplicity.

7. What is upper airway resistance syndrome (UARS)?

Upper airway resistance syndrome (UARS) is a form of OSA where the upper airway obstruction is too subtle to show apneas or hypopneas but still sufficient to cause arousals. The symptoms of UARS and OSA are similar; and they are often collectively called obstructive sleep apnea syndrome (OSAS) or, more accurately, obstructive sleep apnea-hypopnea syndrome (OSAHS).

8. What does a PSG show in case of UARS?

The sleep study usually shows increased number of arousals, but the AHI is <5 since the degree of airway narrowing generally does not meet the criteria for apneas or hypopneas. Many conditions other than UARS also show increase in arousals, e.g., pain, reflux, etc. Definite diagnosis requires demonstration of widely fluctuating intrathoracic pressure with respiration, equipment for which is not routinely available in most clinical sleep laboratories. For this reason, UARS can be suspected but not confirmed on most PSGs, and clinical correlation with history and examination is very important.

One practical way to demonstrate UARS is to show subjective and/or objective improvement with CPAP, either during a titration study in the laboratory or with a home CPAP trial. Improvement does not automatically mean that CPAP is required—it just means UARS is probably present and can be treated with CPAP or other methods used for classic OSA, depending upon the severity of symptoms.

9. What is obesity-hypoventilation syndrome (OHS)?

OHS consists of obesity, often severe, associated with a reduced respiratory drive producing hypoventilation and resultant low oxygen and high carbon dioxide levels in the blood. The hypoventilation is more severe during sleep. The term "Pickwickian syndrome" has been used to describe OHS.

Most (but not all) patients with OHS also have OSA, and the daytime somnolence is due to a combination of disrupted night sleep and carbon dioxide retention.

10. How is OHS different from OSA?

OHS has been considered an extreme form of OSA, but this is an oversimplification since there are fundamental differences in pathophysiology between the two conditions.

- Although OSA is usually seen in obese people, a significant proportion of OSA occurs even in nonobese persons. Obesity, by definition, is always present in OHS.

- In classical OSA, there is no carbon dioxide retention during the day whereas this is a cardinal feature of OHS.

- OSA rarely leads to pulmonary hypertension—this is seen much more commonly with OHS.

11. How is snoring related to OSA?

Snoring is basically noisy breathing during sleep, the sound arising either due to vibration of pharyngeal soft tissues and/or due to turbulent passage of air through the nose. Snoring indicates some degree of air turbulence and *may* be associated with OSA, but this is not always the case. Most people with OSA snore, but only a minority of snorers have clinically significant OSA. Snoring without clinically significant apnea is known as primary snoring.

12. Is snoring alone an indication for a PSG?

No. Snoring is very common in adults, and if there are no other features to suggest sleep apnea, it is not an indication for a PSG since the chances of finding significant apnea are very low. However, snoring should be regarded as a "red flag", especially if it is loud. If snoring is present with symptoms such as excessive somnolence or fatigue or with comorbidities such as hypertension or ischemic heart disease, it is reasonable to consider a PSG since it could potentially influence treatment.

13. How common is OSA?

In adults, symptomatic OSA, i.e., an AHI of 5 or more with symptoms, is reportedly present in 4% of men and 2% of women. If only an AHI of 5 or more is considered (with or without symptoms), the incidence is much higher (24% of men and 9% of women). There is a variation with age (higher in older people) and with ethnicity (higher in African Americans and Asians).

OSA is therefore at least as common as diabetes mellitus and asthma. The steady increase in the prevalence of obesity will likely result in OSA becoming even more common in the future.

14. What are the common risk factors for OSA?

The most important risk factor is obesity and the overweight state. A body mass index (BMI) between 25 and 30 defines the overweight state and >30 defines obesity. Increased neck circumference (>17 inches in men, >16 inches in women) has been associated with increased risk of OSA.

Other risk factors include male gender, increasing age, postmenopausal state, anatomic conditions (e.g., adenotonsillar enlargement, micrognathia, retrognathia, macroglossia, craniofacial abnormalities, deviated nasal septum, nasal congestion, etc.), endocrine disorders (e.g., hypothyroidism and hyperpituitarism), and family history.

Smoking irritates the airway, causing congestion and narrowing of the lumen, thus worsening OSA. Alcohol and sedatives also tend to worsen the severity of apnea (see question 15).

In children, adenotonsillar enlargement is the most important risk factor.

15. How do alcohol and sedatives affect sleep apnea?

Alcohol and sedatives are commonly used as sleeping aids. However, in the presence of sleep apnea, they can actually make matters worse. Both alcohol and sedatives increase the laxity of the upper airway, making it more collapsible. They also increase the arousal threshold, thus tending to prolong apneas. The net effect is increase in the risk and severity of apnea.

Alcohol also has the effect of fragmenting sleep later in the night, adding to the nonrestful effect that apnea can produce.

16. What is the effect of sleep deprivation on sleep apnea?

Anecdotally, some patients with OSA report less snoring and better quality sleep over time, without specific interventions for apnea. A possible explanation is that sleep deprivation diminishes the hypoxic and hypercapnic ventilatory drive to breathe, producing apnea, which improves when the sleep deprivation is eliminated. Patients should therefore be advised about optimal sleep hygiene if there is a suggestion of sleep deprivation on history, even though current-day lifestyles and work pressures often make this difficult to follow.

17. What is the magnitude of undiagnosed sleep apnea?

Despite improved awareness and the knowledge that sleep apnea is associated with significant morbidity and mortality, the majority of patients with this very treatable condition are undiagnosed or are diagnosed very late in the course of the condition. It is estimated that at least 75% of cases of severe sleep apnea are undiagnosed.

18. What are the main consequences of OSA?

These may be divided into two categories:

a. *Poor sleep quality.* This is a direct effect of repeated apneas resulting in multiple arousals at night (without necessarily fully waking the patient).

The symptoms include excessive daytime somnolence, fatigue, morning headaches, irritability, sexual dysfunction, and features mimicking a mood disorder. Excessive daytime somnolence has received a lot of attention, especially in the lay press, since it predisposes to increased number of traffic accidents. Children can present with atypical symptoms, e.g., behavioural problems and paradoxical hyperactivity.

Most of these symptoms are the direct result of disrupted nighttime sleep, but they are not specific for sleep apnea and can occur with many other conditions. For example, the most common cause of excessive somnolence is not sleep apnea but insufficient sleep.

b. *Associated medical conditions.* These include hypertension, coronary artery disease, congestive heart failure, cerebrovascular disease, diabetes mellitus, and some other conditions, the list of which continues to grow (see below). Some of these conditions are discussed in more detail in section 3. Cardiovascular complications are more likely if the patient has moderate to severe apnea. These comorbidities are partly the result of the apnea itself and partly due to common risk factors such as obesity.

Sleep apnea may be associated with pulmonary artery hypertension, especially in people who have the obesity hypoventilation syndrome (OHS). Other associations described with sleep apnea include gout and liver damage. Higher incidence of sleep apnea has also been reported with several endocrine conditions apart from diabetes, e.g., hypothyroidism and hyperpituitarism.

19. How does sleep apnea usually come to medical attention?

Patients are usually suspected of having sleep apnea because of one or more of the following:

- A direct history of observed snoring and apneas

- The results of poor sleep quality (excessive daytime somnolence, fatigue, etc.)

- Associated medical conditions (hypertension, coronary artery disease, etc.)

Often, features from more than one category are present. Health care providers should be vigilant about the possibility of sleep apnea in people with conditions known to be associated with this condition, even if symptoms directly related to sleep apnea are not present.

20. Are symptoms a good indicator of the severity of apnea?

Although the trend is increased symptoms with increased severity, symptoms correlate only roughly with severity. It is not unusual for someone with mild apnea to be very symptomatic (snoring, somnolence, fatigue, etc.) whereas severe apnea may sometimes be associated with practically no symptoms. This is probably partly because patients may minimize or maximize their symptoms, partly because the symptoms are nonspecific and hard to quantify, and partly because the definition of severity based on the AHI is imperfect.

The decision to treat apnea should therefore be made after taking into account the whole clinical picture (symptoms, risk of comorbidities, PSG report, etc.).

21. What is positional apnea?

OSA is usually worse in the supine position, mainly because the tongue falls back with gravity, aggravating the preexisting upper airway obstruction. In some people, apnea is noted in the supine position but not in the nonsupine position. Strictly speaking, positional apnea is diagnosed when the AHI is elevated in the supine position but not in the nonsupine position. There is evidence to suggest that with OSA, the greater the BMI, the less likely it is to be positional.

In theory, positional apnea can be controlled by avoiding supine sleep (see question 22), but this is not always effective or practical, and other forms of treatment may be required.

22. What is positional training/supine avoidance?

This is a technique used for treating positional apnea. The basic idea is to make it uncomfortable or inconvenient to sleep in the supine position, e.g., attaching a tennis balls or a similar object to the back of the night shirt (sleep ball) or using a body pillow to prevent rolling over on the back during sleep.

After a while, some patients become "trained" to sleep in the lateral position and do not need the physical reminder.

Obviously, this technique is useful only for positional apnea (or apnea that is predominantly positional)—it cannot be expected to work if there is no significant difference in the severity of apnea between supine and nonsupine positions.

23. Can sleeping in the "propped up" position affect sleep apnea?

Elevation of the head and trunk to 30-60 degrees has been shown to improve sleep apnea in some cases. This position is usually not evaluated during most PSGs, and the degree of improvement and percentage of patients with OSA that would benefit from this position is uncertain.

The "propped up" sleeping position is part of conservative treatment for CHF, treatment of which can indirectly help CSA-CSR.

24. How is OSA treated in adults?

Conservative measures for treatment of OSA include weight loss, avoiding alcohol close to bedtime, avoiding sedatives, smoking cessation, avoiding supine sleep (in positional apnea), and sleeping with the head and trunk elevated. These measures by themselves can often be sufficient to treat mild apnea. Not all of these measures will apply to every patient.

For moderate to severe apnea, additional treatment is usually required. Such additional treatment includes CPAP or its variations such as bilevel positive pressure (BiPAP), oral appliances or surgery such as uvulopharyngopalatoplasty (UPPP). Treatment should be tailored to the specific patient and sometimes a combination of methods is required.

OSA should not only be treated on the basis of the severity noted on the PSG but after taking into account the severity of symptoms, comorbidities, occupation, etc.

25. How does CPAP work?

CPAP works mainly by splinting open the upper airway (Figure 2).

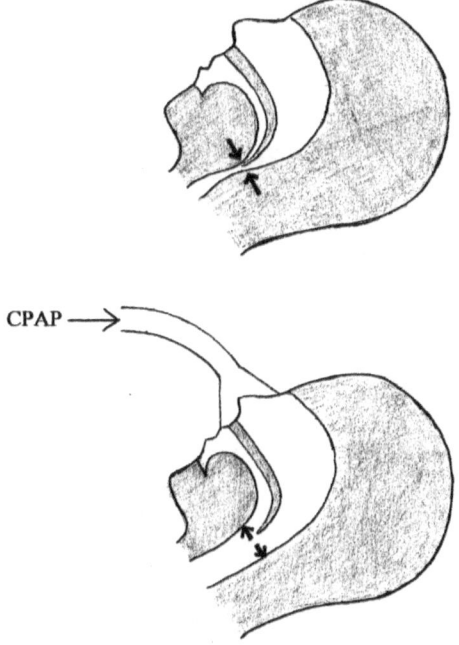

FIGURE 2. EFFECT OF CPAP ON UPPER AIRWAY

Other possible effects include increase in pharyngeal dilator muscle activity, increase in functional residual capacity, and reduction in cardiac afterload. The equipment consists of an air compressor that supplies air at a positive pressure, usually between 4 and 20 cm of water, which is fixed throughout the respiratory cycle. The positive pressure is delivered to the upper airway by means of a hose and nasal or oronasal mask (also called interface) and acts as an air splint, holding the upper airway open, thus relieving the obstruction that would otherwise cause snoring and OSA.

CPAP is the treatment of choice for moderate to severe apnea since other methods are less reliable in that situation. CPAP can also be used for mild apnea if the symptoms are sufficiently severe or if the patient specifically wishes to use it.

Usually, there is no need for supplemental oxygen, but this can be added to CPAP if it is specifically indicated for hypoxemia.

Figure 3 shows a typical CPAP set-up.

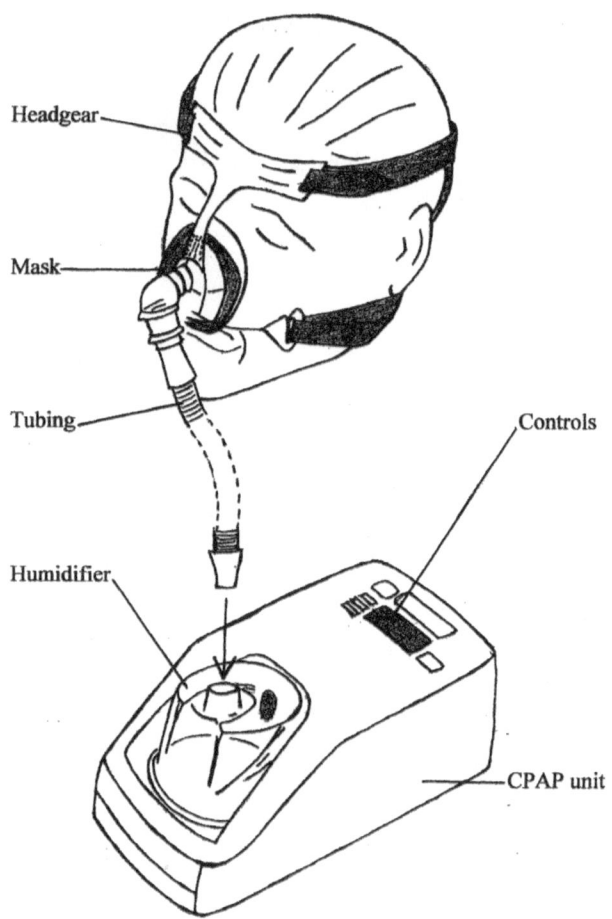

Headgear

Mask

Tubing

Controls

Humidifier

CPAP unit

FIGURE 3. TYPICAL CPAP SET-UP

26. How effective is CPAP for OSA?

CPAP is almost universally effective for OSA, provided the pressure is optimal and the patient is able to tolerate it. This is because it basically eliminates the mechanical reason behind OSA, i.e., upper airway obstruction. Noncompliance is the major reason for CPAP being less effective than it should be (see questions 27 and 28).

27. What is the long-term compliance rate for CPAP?

About 2 out of 3 patients with OSA are still using CPAP after 5 years as reported on long-term follow-up. However, actual usage varies and many patients do not use CPAP throughout the night. A minimum of 4 hours of use per night 5 nights a week has been considered acceptable, but this is an arbitrary definition of compliance. It has been estimated that probably only 50-60% of patients meet this definition.

Long-term use of CPAP by patients is limited by patient motivation, the need to use it consistently, discomfort, and cost of replacement parts, among other factors. The patient's perception of benefit seems to be the most consistent predictor of compliance. Patients reporting problems during the initial CPAP titration study are less likely to use it regularly on a long-term basis.

28. What are the adverse effects of CPAP?

Adverse effects include a feeling of claustrophobia, nasal congestion, oronasal dryness, epistaxis, sinus discomfort, and uncomfortable air leaks between mask and face. Other side effects include skin abrasion/rash from the interface, aerophagy, and difficulty exhaling, particularly at higher pressures. Added to the modest inconvenience of having to use it regularly, these problems result in difficulty adapting to CPAP therapy.

29. What is autotitrating CPAP?

An autotitrating CPAP device, as the name suggests, is a self-adjusting device that detects upper airway obstruction and changes the CPAP level appropriately according to a preset algorithm. In theory, it should avoid excessive pressure sometimes associated with fixed CPAP units and should therefore improve compliance. However, the evidence for improved compliance is conflicting.

Autotitrating CPAP units are being used for unattended home CPAP titrations (see question 62).

30. How is CSA treated?

CSA is best treated by treating the underlying condition, e.g., congestive heart failure. Reducing or eliminating sedatives can be beneficial. CPAP can be effective for CSA though not as consistently as for OSA. CPAP is commonly used when CSA coexists with OSA. There is some evidence that CSA responds better to CPAP when it is present with predominant OSA or when it occurs in association with CHF.

Other methods of treatment include oxygen, bilevel positive pressure (BiPAP), and adaptive servo-ventilation (ASV), with varying degrees of success. BiPAP and ASV are mentioned in more detail later.

Some patients benefit from respiratory stimulant medication, e.g., acetazolamide (see question 35).

Rarely, diaphragmatic pacing may be indicated for apnea resulting from neurologic lesions above the second or third cervical level.

31. What is "complex" sleep apnea?

This is a relatively new term, referring to a situation where a patient with OSA develops CSA during a CPAP titration study. In fact, it may be considered a complication of using CPAP. Some authorities consider it the result of excessively rapid upward titration of CPAP rather than a true clinical entity. Knowledge about this phenomenon is still evolving. Initially, it was believed to be present in about 15% of all people with OSA, but other authorities have found it to be much less common.

In some patients with complex sleep apnea (which, by definition, is found during CPAP titration), the condition disappears with regular CPAP use, and CPAP can be used with benefit on a long-term basis. Bilevel positive pressure (BiPAP) has been tried but with limited and variable success. Some patients require adaptive servo-ventilation (ASV), which is described below.

32. What is bilevel positive airway pressure (BiPAP)?

BiPAP involves using two levels of pressure instead of a single level as in CPAP. Like CPAP, it provides an "air splint", but it provides a relatively higher pressure during inspiration (IPAP) and a relatively lower pressure during expiration (EPAP). The result is that patients do not have to breathe against a high pressure when they are exhaling. The main use of BiPAP in sleep apnea has been for patients requiring high levels of CPAP (15 cm of water or more) where the lower pressure during expiration is more comfortable without allowing upper airway closure. This should result in better compliance with treatment, but in fact BiPAP has not been shown to improve compliance significantly compared to CPAP.

More recently, BiPAP has been used for the newly described complex sleep apnea although this role may be taken over by adaptive servo-ventilation (ASV)—see question 33.

33. What is adaptive servo-ventilation (ASV)?

ASV is a relatively new form of noninvasive ventilation. The ASV unit basically monitors the patient's respiration on a breath-by-breath basis according to a preset algorithm and provides pressure support appropriately as and when required. It can be used for CSA and may be the treatment of choice for complex sleep apnea although treatment for the latter condition is still evolving.

So far, cost has been a major barrier to the use of ASV, at least in Canada.

34. What is the role of supplemental oxygen in the treatment of apnea?

Supplemental oxygen, when used by itself to prevent desaturations in OSA, has been found to have variable effects. It can reduce desaturations but can also prolong the apneas. For this reason, its use as sole therapy in OSAS is limited and requires careful monitoring. When it is used for OSA, it is usually in association with CPAP when positive pressure is not sufficient to maintain adequate oxygen saturation.

CSA-CSR sometimes responds to oxygen therapy alone.

35. What drugs can be used for sleep apnea?

Protriptyline, a tricyclic antidepressant, increases upper airway dilator muscle tone and reduces REM sleep, thus potentially improving OSA.

Unfortunately, side effects have limited its use. Medroxyprogesterone has been tried due to its respiratory stimulant effect but with minimal, if any, benefit. Acetazolamide is sometimes used for CSA because of its effect of producing metabolic acidosis, thereby stimulating respiration centrally. Other drugs have been used because of their respiratory stimulant effects; but in general, drug therapy has been disappointing for the treatment of sleep apnea, especially OSA.

Sometimes, stimulants are used to combat dangerous daytime somnolence due to OSA if it persists despite treatment with CPAP. Amphetamines have been traditionally used, but they have significant side effects. Caffeine is very commonly used as a stimulant, mostly in the form of caffeine-containing beverages; this may be the most commonly used stimulant worldwide. Modafinil is a relatively new stimulant with fewer side effects and can be used for residual somnolence despite CPAP therapy.

The use of stimulants for sleep apnea is not universally accepted since they do not address the primary problem of apnea but only attempt to relieve one of its consequences (somnolence).

36. How do oral appliances work?

Oral appliances usually work by either moving the jaw forward (jaw repositioning devices) or repositioning the tongue (tongue repositioning devices). Different types of each kind are available, but the basic mechanism of action is increasing upper airway patency and preventing collapse. Oral appliances are effective only in mild to moderate apnea, being either ineffective or only partially effective in severe apnea. Jaw pain and tooth discomfort are some of the known side effects of oral appliances.

Referral to a dentist or denturist with experience in this field is recommended if this treatment is being considered.

37. What surgical options are available for OSA?

The most common surgical procedure for OSA in adults is uvulopalatopharyngoplasty (UPPP), but it is of limited efficacy for OSA. Success rates for selected patients are reported to be around 50% for OSA although higher success rates have been reported for primary snoring. UPPP results in reduction of soft palatal/pharyngeal tissue, which is responsible for vibration causing snoring. Sometimes, UPPP is used in conjunction with other operations, such as genioglossus advancement or hyoid suspension. Alteration of speech and velopalatal insufficiency are recognized complications of UPPP.

Like dental appliances, UPPP is most useful for mild to moderate OSA and works best in conjunction with weight loss. Also like dental appliances, UPPP is unlikely to control severe apnea completely. Laser-assisted uvuloplasty (LAUP) is a variation of UPPP but not as well studied.

Adenotonsillectomy is an option when there is significant adenoidal or tonsillar enlargement. This is most commonly seen in children (see question 38).

Occasionally, an anatomic maxillomandibular anomaly is present (e.g., micrognathia or retrognathia), surgical correction of which may relieve the apnea. Other surgical procedures such as tongue base surgery are occasionally useful.

Tracheostomy is very effective in treating OSA by bypassing the obstruction. Once the only treatment available for severe apnea, it is now rarely used and is usually reserved for life-threatening apnea that cannot be treated in any other manner.

38. How is OSA treated in children?

In children, adenotonsillar enlargement is the most common cause of OSA, and adenotonsillectomy is therefore the treatment of choice. This procedure can also be performed in the minority of adults who have significant adenotonsillar enlargement and can be combined with UPPP. Consultation with an ENT specialist is recommended in such cases.

Further details on treatment of OSA in the pediatric population are outside the scope of this book.

39. How does severity of apnea correlate with morbidity and mortality?

Patients with moderate to severe apnea are at increased risk of cardiovascular conditions, including hypertension, coronary artery disease, and stroke, which are associated with increased morbidity and mortality. There is also a recently described association with type 2 diabetes mellitus.

Recent evidence suggests that increasing severity of sleep apnea is associated with significant increase in all-cause mortality.

40. Why is it important to treat OSA?

Sleep apnea is treated for two main reasons:

- To relieve symptoms such as sleepiness and fatigue

- To reduce the risk of comorbidity

The decision is straightforward when both problems are present and the patient has moderate to severe apnea—treatment is required. The decision is not so easy when no symptoms are present or there is a low risk of comorbidities. This is particularly so when the severity of the apnea is also in question.

41. How does clinical judgment influence treatment of OSA?

Clinical judgment is always required when deciding on treatment; the result of a PSG is not sufficient. For example, if the AHI is only 10, treatment may not be necessary if the patient is an asymptomatic nonobese young woman. In fact, one would even question the reason for doing a PSG in such an individual. On the other hand, with the same AHI, treatment is probably required in a morbidly obese patient (BMI >40) who has hypertension, ischemic heart disease, or cerebrovascular disease, even if there are no symptoms.

Many patients will fall in between these two examples, and the decision to treat and the actual choice of therapy require clinical judgment.

SECTION 2

SLEEP STUDIES AND RELATED TESTS FOR APNEA

42. What is a sleep study (PSG)?

A sleep study or polysomnogram (PSG) is a technique involving the recording of multiple simultaneous physiologic characteristics acquired from a subject during overnight sleep in a sleep laboratory (see question 43). The data is collected, analyzed, and compared with data from normal subjects to determine whether or not a sleep disorder is present.

Unlike many other clinical tests, the PSG was initially designed as a research tool and only later applied to clinical practice. The PSG has never been validated as a clinical tool but is nevertheless used as such for lack of a better method.

Originally, sleep studies were recorded on paper. Modern computer technology has made recording simpler, but data collection is still very labor-intensive. Sleep from the entire night is broken up into 30-second periods called epochs, each of which is manually examined by the sleep technician to determine the stage of sleep and record physiological data (scoring). The study is then interpreted by a physician with expertise in the area. The process is time-consuming and is one reason for the lag time between performing the study and obtaining the result.

43. *What information can a PSG provide?*

Commonly recorded physiologic data includes EEG, eye movements, EKG, respiratory effort, nasal-oral airflow, oximetry, and muscle tone. Additional information can be obtained by sound recording (snoring) and video recording to detect abnormal motor activity during sleep. The different stages of sleep are determined from the EEG, muscle tone, and eye movements.

The vast majority of PSGs done in clinical practice are for suspected sleep apnea or for titration of CPAP, but PSGs can be tailored to look for certain other specific conditions (see below). It is therefore important to include relevant clinical information with the referral.

44. *What information can a PSG* **not** *provide?*

PSGs are designed to detect and record physiologic phenomena but not subjective experiences, which cannot be picked up as signals. Pain, discomfort, emotional states, dream content, etc. cannot be recorded with current technology; and a PSG is not indicated for these conditions. *It is important to appreciate this point in order to avoid subjecting people to unnecessary PSGs.*

A PSG is generally not indicated for insomnia since it would be unlikely to show any characteristic signal pattern and the result would not add anything to management.

PSGs should be performed with the understanding that sleep in the laboratory is usually not representative of sleep in more "natural" surroundings at home. Therefore, they should not be ordered just to check the sleep quality.

45. *What are the common indications for a PSG?*

The most common indication for a PSG is suspected sleep apnea (so-called diagnostic PSG). A PSG can provide information about the presence and severity of sleep apnea even though the technology is not perfect. PSGs are also indicated for the titration of CPAP (so-called CPAP titration studies) so that an optimal CPAP level can be prescribed for patients known to have sleep apnea. The vast majority of PSGs are done for these two indications.

PSGs are ordered for other conditions such as periodic limb movements and nocturnal seizures, but their use in these situations is limited (see questions 55 and 58).

46. How is sleep apnea diagnosed and differentiated on a PSG?

OSA is due to mechanical narrowing and obstruction of the upper airway, with respiratory effort being intact. CSA is due to absence of respiratory effort, with the upper airway playing no role. Therefore, on the PSG, diagnosis of OSA requires demonstration of apnea with intact respiratory effort whereas diagnosis of CSA requires demonstration of apnea without respiratory effort (Figure 1).

When the term "sleep apnea" is used, it generally refers to OSA although strictly speaking, one should specify whether it is obstructive or central.

47. What are the other (infrequent) indications for a PSG?

Patients are sometimes referred to the sleep laboratory for suspected narcolepsy, a condition characterized by somnolence, cataplexy, hypnagogic/ hypnopompic hallucinations, and sleep paralysis (in varying combinations). This condition requires a *daytime* test called multiple sleep latency test (MSLT) to assess the level of sleepiness and also to check for rapid onset of REM sleep—a characteristic of narcolepsy. This test requires a PSG during the preceding night to rule out other sleep problems even though it is not directly required to diagnose narcolepsy.

Rarely, a PSG may be ordered to look for abnormal movements or behaviour in sleep (parasomnias). One such condition is REM behaviour disorder (RBD), the hallmark of which is abnormally high muscle tone during REM sleep. Similarly, PSGs may be occasionally ordered for other rare conditions. In such cases, it is very important to supply the sleep laboratory with details about what is being looked for, so that the study can be modified appropriately.

48. How good is a PSG for detecting sleep apnea?

Despite its limitations, the overnight PSG is the best tool available for diagnosing OSA or CSA. False positives are rare, but false negatives are common, i.e., a PSG can underestimate or even miss significant apnea. This may be due to

- lack of supine sleep, which is usually associated with increased severity of OSA;

- suboptimal sleep quality during the study, especially lack of REM sleep (during which OSA is usually worse);

- omission of alcohol or sedatives before the study, if the patient is regularly using these substances;

- technical problems with signals, resulting in missing apneas or hypopneas.

In other words, a PSG can almost always rule in sleep apnea but may not rule it out.

49. What information about sleep apnea can be obtained from a PSG?

A diagnostic PSG can confirm the presence of sleep apnea and can categorize it as obstructive or central. It can also give an idea about its severity although the methodology is far from perfect. The apnea-hypopnea index (AHI) gives a rough idea about the severity, but the true severity probably also depends on other factors such as degree of oxygen desaturation and the autonomic response to the apneas. An ideal number expressing the severity of the apnea is not available.

When performed for titration of CPAP, PSGs can help to determine an optimal level of CPAP for each individual patient. Such a study involves monitoring the patient as would be required for a diagnostic PSG with the addition of CPAP, which is adjusted during the study. Again, the technology is not perfect; but some idea can be obtained about the optimal CPAP level, which can be modified later if required.

50. What will a PSG add to my clinical suspicion of sleep apnea?

Like any diagnostic study, the value of a PSG depends upon the pretest probability. Before ordering a PSG, as for any diagnostic test, the clinician should assess the likelihood of the condition being present. Ordering a PSG when there is little or no likelihood of sleep apnea can produce confusing results if the test is positive. For example, if a nonobese young woman with no symptoms and no cardiovascular risk factors undergoes a PSG and the result indicates mild apnea, the report may not be clinically relevant; and there is no evidence that treatment will be beneficial. On the other hand, a symptomatic hypertensive obese middle-aged man has a much higher pretest probability of having OSA. In this case, it is appropriate to confirm the diagnosis and severity of the apnea with a PSG.

51. How is the severity of apnea assessed on a PSG?

The severity of sleep apnea is usually determined by the AHI. An AHI of <5 is considered normal for adults. The threshold is lower for children although reliable normal values are not available. In adults, an AHI of 5-15 is considered mild, 15-30 moderate, and >30 severe. However, this is just a "rule of thumb", and other factors such as degree of oxygen desaturation also need to be considered. For example, desaturation down to 70% should indicate more severe apnea than desaturation to only 85%, even if the AHI is the same in both cases. Currently, there is no good method available to reflect all the variables that contribute to the severity of apnea.

Patients often do not sleep well in the artificial setting of a sleep laboratory, making it difficult to apply the results to sleep at home. Sometimes, mild sleep apnea in the laboratory is actually an underestimation because of poor sleep quality and absence of certain stages, e.g., REM sleep, during which OSA is usually worse. Clinical correlation should be applied when applying the results of a PSG.

52. Why is a PSG carried out overnight instead of during a single daytime nap?

Overnight sleep usually includes periods of REM sleep, the stage in which sleep apnea is most severe. It is unusual to capture REM sleep during a single daytime nap. Since the main indication for a PSG is suspected sleep apnea, overnight sleep is generally preferred.

Exceptions are made for patients whose sleep pattern involves sleeping in the day and keeping awake at night, e.g., people on night shifts. In such cases, daytime PSGs are arranged, but the duration is kept long enough to include some REM sleep.

53. What is a "split night" study?

A split night study is basically a diagnostic PSG and a CPAP titration study combined into a single study during one night. Instead of doing a diagnostic PSG on one night and a CPAP titration on another, a split night study includes the diagnostic portion in the first part of the night and CPAP titration in the second part. There are some drawbacks with this process. The time available for each of the diagnostic and CPAP titration parts is very limited, sometimes resulting in insufficient data. Also, one is comparing the first part of the night with the second even though they differ in the composition of sleep stages (slow-wave sleep predominates in the first part and REM sleep in the second).

Despite the disadvantages, the benefits in terms of cost, convenience, and speed of results makes a split night study a practical option in some situations.

54. What is the role of a PSG in the diagnosis of restless legs syndrome (RLS)?

RLS is a condition characterized by symptoms of discomfort in the legs, typically occurring late in the day. This condition can result in difficulty in falling asleep (initial insomnia), but by definition, it does not occur *during* sleep. The diagnosis is purely on the basis of history and exclusion of other conditions. Thus a PSG has no role to play in the diagnosis of RLS except to look for periodic limb movement disorder (PLMD), which often coexists with RLS (but see question 55).

55. Is suspected PLMD an indication for a PSG?

Opinion is divided on this issue. Some clinicians prefer to order a PSG to detect the movements during sleep. Others prefer to rely on history and response to treatment. PLMD often occurs with RLS but can occur by itself.

PLMD can be detected on a PSG, but the movements can be difficult to distinguish from movements due to other causes such as respiratory arousals. The severity of the condition can vary from night to night and may be missed on a single PSG. For these reasons, some clinicians do not believe a PSG is helpful in making this diagnosis.

56. Is insomnia an indication for a PSG?

Transient/short-term insomnia is, by definition, short-lived and does not require a PSG.

Generally, chronic insomnia is *not* an indication for a sleep study. Most cases of insomnia result from psychological, neurological, or medical conditions that can be diagnosed by history, examination, and tests other than a PSG. Insomnia by itself is unlikely to be associated with any findings on a PSG that will alter the treatment.

Occasionally, PSGs are done in patients with chronic insomnia, but these are to detect coexisting problems or in the uncommon case of sleep apnea being suspected as the cause of insomnia. A practical problem is that patients with insomnia are, by definition, poor sleepers; and the PSG is therefore more likely to be nondiagnostic.

57. Is sleepwalking an indication for a PSG?

Not usually. Sleepwalking (somnambulism) occurs commonly in children and occasionally in adults. It occurs more commonly in slow-wave sleep and is therefore most likely to occur in the first half of the night. It can usually be diagnosed by history alone, sometimes requiring tests to rule out underlying medical conditions. A PSG is only occasionally required if there is confusion about the diagnosis or other conditions mimicking sleepwalking cannot be ruled out.

58. What is the role of a PSG for seizures?

The utility of PSGs for seizures is limited since most cases can be diagnosed by history and daytime investigations. Only 10% of all seizures occur exclusively at night. Nevertheless, suspected nocturnal seizures is one of the indications for a PSG.

Additional head electrodes may be required to increase the diagnostic yield for seizures (so-called seizure montage). Video recording is also useful for picking up seizure activity at night. It is therefore advisable to inform the sleep laboratory that the study is being requested for nocturnal seizures.

59. What is the role of unattended (home) sleep studies?

Home studies are screening tools and can indicate the likelihood of the presence and severity of apnea. They can be useful to decide whether or not a patient should be investigated further with a formal PSG. Very occasionally, if symptoms are typical and a home study indicates a high probability of apnea, treatment may be initiated without a formal PSG in the interest of time.

Limited validation data is available for unattended home studies and currently a PSG performed in a sleep laboratory is the accepted "gold standard" for diagnosis of sleep apnea. However, as demand increases, home studies may be used more frequently in the future.

60. What is the role of home overnight oximetry?

Home overnight oximetry has been used as a screening tool to help decide whether or not to refer the patient for a PSG, but it is of limited value since it is neither sensitive nor specific. Significant apnea can be present without desaturation, e.g., when the duration of apnea is not long enough to produce desaturation. As well, there are other causes for desaturation besides sleep apnea (see question 61).

Significant desaturations at night, when present in conjunction with an appropriate history, are an indication for a formal PSG.

Home oximetry can also be used to follow up patients who are known to desaturate and are using CPAP, to check for adequacy of treatment.

61. Other than sleep apnea, what are the causes of oxygen desaturation at night?

Oxygen saturation during sleep is generally slightly lower than awake values even in normal subjects. In certain conditions, the baseline saturation may be low and drops even lower during sleep. Many pulmonary diseases, e.g., COPD and interstitial lung disease, can cause nocturnal oxygen desaturation. COPD often causes disproportionately severe desaturations in REM sleep due to preexisting problems with a relatively nonmobile and flat diaphragm.

Other causes of nocturnal desaturation include CHF and hypoventilation due to any cause, e.g., sedative/narcotic medication.

62. What is the role of home CPAP titration (autotitration)?

CPAP titration in a sleep laboratory is the "gold standard" for determining the optimal CPAP level. However, this process has obvious drawbacks, e.g., inconvenience to the patient, sleeping in unfamiliar surroundings, limited testing during a single night, government/insurance restrictions on the number of sleep studies, healthcare costs, etc. CPAP titration at home, using an autotitrating device, has been used as a cheaper and more convenient alternative (see question 29).

While nothing can replace attended titration in the laboratory, where a technician is available to troubleshoot if necessary, home autotitration has the advantage of being cheaper and more convenient. It can also be applied over several days, and this may help the patient to get used to CPAP at home.

Home autotitration has been used when formal titration in the laboratory is either impractical, unsuccessful, or refused by the patient. Some physicians prefer home autotitration to formal titration in the laboratory. With the increasing demand for investigations for sleep apnea, home autotitration studies may become more popular in the future, freeing up sleep studies in the laboratory for diagnostic purposes.

SECTION 3

SLEEP APNEA AND SELECTED MEDICAL CONDITIONS

63. *With obesity, how effective is weight loss for OSA?*

Weight loss can be quite effective for sleep apnea. In one study, a 10% weight loss predicted a 26% improvement in the AHI. The problem with weight loss is implementation since it requires a lot of motivation on the part of the patient. Bariatric surgery has become an increasingly common form of weight loss treatment in morbidly obese patients when other measures have been unsuccessful.

Weight loss by itself may be sufficient treatment for mild OSA. Even for moderate to severe OSA, weight loss is complementary when used in combination with other methods. Oral appliances and surgery are generally more effective when combined with weight loss. Even patients on CPAP can sometimes be treated with lower CPAP levels after weight loss.

64. *Since CPAP is so effective for OSA, is weight loss still important?*

In the author's opinion, weight loss has generally been underemphasized as a form of treatment for OSA. When successfully implemented, it is effective for OSA, and it is also a valuable adjunctive measure to other forms of treatment.

Apart from its beneficial effect on OSA, losing weight has other independent health benefits, including better blood pressure control, improved glucose tolerance, reduced risk of certain malignancies, enhanced mobility, and reduced risk of degenerative joint disease. There are also obvious psychological benefits to losing weight.

For these reasons, with few exceptions, weight loss should be recommended when the BMI is significantly elevated.

65. How is sleep apnea related to hypertension?

Systemic hypertension is the medical condition best known to be associated with OSA. Subjects with an AHI of 15 or more (moderate to severe apnea) have a two to threefold risk of hypertension compared to subjects without OSA. The increased risk cannot be explained on the basis of weight, age, gender, body habitus, or smoking. The prevalence of OSA is particularly high in patients with refractory hypertension. Repeated arousals and hypoxemia produce increased catecholamine activity, which is the probable explanation for the increase in blood pressure.

Modest reduction in blood pressure (2-10 mm drop in mean arterial pressure) has been seen following institution of CPAP therapy, with the greatest benefit being noted in severe OSA on effective treatment.

66. How is sleep apnea related to coronary artery disease?

The prevalence of coronary artery disease is higher in OSA than in the general population. In one study, coronary artery disease was present in almost 25% of OSA subjects, especially those with moderate to severe apnea. Also, about one third of patients with CAD appear to have OSA.

OSA is also believed to aggravate preexisting coronary artery disease. Nocturnal ischemic changes on EKG are more common with OSA and can be eliminated with CPAP. Hypoxemia, reoxygenation, and recurrent arterial wall stress during sleep are believed to be the mechanisms by which OSA causes or aggravates CAD.

67. How is sleep apnea related to stroke?

OSA is a risk factor for stroke due to increase in the prevalence of hypertension. Mechanisms similar to those described for coronary artery disease may also be responsible for deleterious effects on the blood vessels, resulting in increased risk of stroke independent of other factors.

Stroke by itself can increase the risk for CSA-CSR if there are bilateral supratentorial lesions causing hypersensitivity to carbon dioxide. Stroke can also disrupt upper airway muscle coordination, increasing the risk of OSA after the event.

68. How is sleep apnea related to CHF?

CHF can be both an effect and a cause of sleep apnea and the relationship is complex. Both CSA and OSA are seen in association with CHF.

OSA has been shown to increase the risk of CHF, likely as a result of increased blood pressure and possibly hypoxemic left ventricular dysfunction.

CHF itself can cause CSA-CSR due to increased arterial circulation time and change in chemoreceptor sensitivity. CHF can also cause OSA by increasing venous congestion, resulting in reduction of the upper airway lumen. Additionally, CSA caused by CHF affects neuromuscular control of the upper airway muscles, raising the risk for OSA.

69. How is sleep apnea related to diabetes mellitus?

OSA has been found to increase the risk of glucose intolerance and type 2 diabetes mellitus. This risk is independent of obesity. The mechanism is believed to be disrupted sleep causing hormonal changes that impair the action of insulin. Some evidence suggests a beneficial effect of CPAP therapy on glucose tolerance.

70. How is sleep apnea related to hypothyroidism?

Hypothyroidism can indirectly predispose to OSA by producing obesity. Deposition of myxedematous tissue and impairment of airway muscles have been suggested as causes of narrowing of the upper airway, but the contributions of such mechanisms is unclear. Some of the symptoms of hypothyroidism, such as fatigue and somnolence, can mimic those of OSA.

Routine screening of all OSA patients for hypothyroidism has not generally been found to be helpful.

71. What special features are seen when sleep apnea coexists with COPD?

Both COPD and sleep apnea are more prevalent with increasing age. With obesity on the rise and the prevalence of COPD being expected to increase in the future, it is only to be expected that sleep apnea and COPD will commonly coexist (so-called overlap syndrome).

COPD causes disproportionately severe desaturation during REM sleep. This tends to aggravate any desaturation occurring with sleep apnea alone. It is thus important to detect the presence of OSA in patients with COPD since supplemental oxygen may be required in addition to CPAP. Some patients may even require noninvasive positive pressure ventilation (NIPPV).

72. How is sleep apnea related to gastroesophageal reflux disease (GERD)?

There is a high incidence of GERD in patients with OSA although the cause and effect relationship is unclear—many patients with OSA are also obese, which increases the risk of GERD. The presence of nocturnal GERD symptoms can worsen the nonrestful sleep already caused by OSA.

Acid suppression is the main treatment for nocturnal GERD, but some data suggests that CPAP therapy provides additional benefits for this condition.

73. Why is it important to detect sleep apnea before administering a general anesthetic?

Central nervous system depressants can aggravate OSA by decreasing the tone of pharyngeal muscles and can reduce the neural drive for respiration, producing central apnea. Preexisting apnea therefore poses increased risk of postoperative respiratory and cardiac complications in patients who receive general anesthesia and postoperative narcotic analgesia or sedation.

OSA patients are also at higher risk of difficult intubation. Loss of airway control after induction of anesthesia is a potential problem in patients with OSA. It is therefore important to be vigilant for these complications in patients known to have OSA and those who are at high risk. Sometimes, this may mean a decision to perform awake intubation. At other times, regional anesthesia may be preferred and the anesthetist usually makes this decision.

Ideally, the severity of the apnea should be known and appropriate treatment initiated before surgery requiring general anesthesia and/or narcotic medication. Depending upon the clinical suspicion of apnea, a preoperative PSG may be required.

CPAP equipment should be available, and postoperative oximetry and cardiac monitoring should be considered for patients known or suspected to have significant OSA.

74. What are the consequences of sleep apnea during pregnancy?

Weight gain and complex hormonal changes can predispose to OSA during pregnancy or can make preexisting OSA worse. However, increase in progesterone has a relatively protective effect against OSA. The presence of OSA poses increased risk of maternal complications, such as preeclampsia, and increased risk of fetal complications, such as low birth weight, prematurity, and (if it is sufficiently severe) fetal complications of hypoxemia. Treatment is therefore required to prevent both maternal and fetal problems.

75. Who should be evaluated for sleep apnea in pregnancy?

The following groups of women should be considered for evaluation for OSA in pregnancy:

- Women who are overweight/obese before pregnancy

- Women who gain excessive weight in pregnancy

- Women who develop new onset of snoring or whose snoring worsens significantly during pregnancy.

A high index of suspicion is required to make the diagnosis of OSA in pregnancy since many of the symptoms of apnea (somnolence, fatigue, etc.) occur as a result of pregnancy itself.

SECTION 4

SELECTED MANAGEMENT ISSUES

76. My patient believes he/she did not sleep well (or did not sleep at all) in the sleep laboratory, and the result of the PSG is therefore meaningless. What should be my response?

Most people do not sleep as well in the sleep laboratory as they do at home. A PSG is not designed to check how they usually sleep but to look for specific conditions such as sleep apnea. Therefore, even if little sleep was achieved, there is a good chance that some useful information will be available.

Some patients have what is known as sleep state misperception, i.e., they grossly underestimate the amount of sleep they get. In these cases, although they may think they did not sleep at all, some sleep may, in fact, have been recorded. It is unusual for no sleep to be recorded during a PSG performed over a whole night.

77. How useful are commercially available nasal breathing strips and specially designed pillows for OSA?

These products basically help to reduce snoring. Nasal breathing strips help by increasing the caliber of the nasal passages during sleep, and they are relatively inexpensive. However, most OSA arises from the pharynx, so the benefit is variable and can be expected to be limited. Specially designed pillows are supposed to help snoring by supporting the neck in particular positions and/or preventing the sleeper from rolling over on the back.

These products may have a role in primary snoring and mild OSA but have not been well studied and are not part of standard recommended therapy for OSA.

78. My patient has severe OSA but denies any symptoms. Should he/she still be treated?

Yes. Moderate to severe OSA should be treated not only for symptomatic improvement but to prevent comorbid conditions, particularly cardiovascular problems. If such problems already exist, treatment becomes more imperative. CPAP is the treatment of choice for moderate to severe OSA since the risk of cardiovascular complications is usually quite high.

Patients are probably more likely to use CPAP if they have symptoms that improve with treatment. If they have no symptoms, compliance can be an issue since no immediate improvement is noted. A frank explanation of the purpose of CPAP and the health risks of untreated sleep apnea may improve compliance. Some patients may need repeated periodic reinforcement of this advice.

79. My patient has just started using CPAP. How soon can he/she expect to notice any benefit?

As mentioned above, there are two main reasons for treating sleep apnea—reduction of risk of comorbid conditions and symptomatic relief. The former is a long-term goal, and immediate benefit is not expected.

Regarding symptomatic relief, the speed of improvement is very variable. Some patients notice improvement the very first night they use CPAP, e.g., after the CPAP titration study in the laboratory. Others take days or weeks, depending upon how quickly they adapt to CPAP. Anecdotally, it appears that the more severe the symptoms, the more dramatic the symptomatic benefit (provided CPAP is used as directed and the patient adapts to the treatment). Some patients require a lot of motivation.

Some patients do not adapt well to CPAP, and it is then important to identify the reason and correct it if possible (see question 80).

80. What can be done for my patient with severe OSA who refuses (or cannot adapt to) CPAP?

The patient should be advised that CPAP is the treatment of choice because severe apnea increases the risk of symptoms and comorbidities. Knowing the importance of treatment and the risks of no treatment can be a strong motivating factor.

In case of discomfort with CPAP, changes can be made in the humidity of the inspired air, in the mask used, or in the pressure. Features such as ramping can sometimes help patients tolerate CPAP better. CPAP suppliers can be very helpful in these matters and can usually work closely with the patient. Setting the pressure slightly lower than recommended is sometimes useful; the pressure can be increased after the patient has adapted to CPAP.

Sometimes, modifications to the way positive pressure is delivered can make a difference. An autotitrating unit (see questions 29 and 62) may be more acceptable since the machine is supposed to adjust the pressure based on requirement (though this mechanism is not without drawbacks). Sometimes, using CPAP with a modification called expiratory pressure relief (EPR) may be helpful by lowering the pressure slightly during expiration without compromising airway patency. Occasionally, a bilevel (BiPAP) unit may be required, especially if the CPAP level is quite high (e.g., 15 cm of water or above), in which case again, the lower pressure during expiration may provide sufficient comfort to allow regular use of the device.

Patients with OSA should be encouraged to explore various options before rejecting CPAP and its modifications altogether, especially if the apnea is severe.

81. My patient has severe OSA but is unable to adapt to CPAP despite the measures mentioned above. What other options are available?

Despite all attempts, some patients will refuse or be unable to use CPAP. Oral appliances and/or ENT procedures such as UPPP can then be considered, recognizing that these methods will likely not control moderate to severe apnea completely (some treatment is better than no treatment).

Lifestyle measures, such as weight loss, cessation of smoking, avoiding alcohol before bedtime and (with positional apnea) avoiding supine sleep, become more important when CPAP cannot be used.

In rare cases, when all other methods fail, patients with severe, life-threatening OSA may require tracheostomy, which bypasses the site of upper airway obstruction. This treatment is very effective but is now rarely used and considered only as a last resort.

82. My patient is using CPAP but not feeling better. What is the explanation?

Noncompliance is an important cause for lack of symptomatic benefit with CPAP. Compliance can be checked in several ways—direct questioning of the patient, collateral information from the bed partner, card readers for the CPAP units, etc.

If there were few or no symptoms before treatment, the improvement may not be noticeable. Another reason could be the initial adaptation period—the inconvenience and discomfort of using CPAP may outweigh the symptomatic improvement. The CPAP supplier can be a valuable resource in this situation, and good organizations work with patients to ensure the highest possible level of comfort with the equipment.

The pressure setting may not be optimal for the patient, even if this is based on the results of a titration study. Adjusting the pressure upward or downward may be all that is required. Patients can sometimes tell if the pressure is too high or too low.

Symptoms like somnolence, fatigue, and irritability are nonspecific and may not necessarily be due to sleep apnea. CPAP can be expected to help symptoms due to sleep apnea, but not those due to other conditions, even if the symptoms are similar. For example, if poor sleeping habits, insufficient sleep, depression, shift work, or chronic pain are responsible for daytime sleepiness, these will not be corrected with CPAP. Such conditions should be sought out by history and corrected if possible.

Permanent hypoxemic brain damage from previous untreated OSA can result in persistent sleepiness despite CPAP therapy.

83. My patient is on CPAP. Will he/she eventually be able to do without it?

CPAP is meant to control apnea while it is being used—it is not a "cure" in the strict sense. Generally, patients on CPAP require it indefinitely unless mechanical factors change, e.g., with considerable weight loss, ENT surgery, or surgical correction of craniofacial abnormalities. Even with these measures, some residual apnea may remain; and if this is sufficiently severe, CPAP may be required. It is therefore unwise to promise patients that they will not need CPAP in the future.

84. My patient is using CPAP but only intermittently. What should be my advice?

For maximum benefit, patients should use CPAP every time they sleep and throughout the sleep period. Using it intermittently or only for part of the night just means they will get less than optimal benefit from it, both in terms of symptoms and prevention of complications. CPAP works only while it is being used, and less-than-compliant patients should be reminded about this fact. A minimum of 4 hours of CPAP for 5 nights a week has been considered acceptable; but generally, the more hours of use, the greater the benefit from CPAP.

85. My patient is going for bariatric surgery. Does he/she need a preoperative PSG?

Some bariatric centres routinely require PSGs before surgery. Others require PSGs if the patient's preoperative questionnaire suggests sleep apnea. Either way, demand for PSGs before bariatric surgery is becoming very common. The rationale for preoperative PSGs before such surgery are as follows:

- Morbid obesity, the indication for bariatric surgery, is very commonly associated with sleep apnea. It has been found that most patients referred for bariatric surgery have sleep apnea whether or not it was previously suspected.

- Preoperative detection of apnea and its treatment is important from the perioperative management point of view (see question 73).

- A preoperative PSG can serve as a baseline for postoperative evaluation to check for improvement in the apnea.

86. My patient has lost a lot of weight since he/she was first diagnosed with OSA and put on CPAP. Should he/she be reevaluated for apnea?

Any intervention that can potentially improve or eliminate apnea should lead to a reevaluation of the severity of the apnea. Patients who initially had OSA and have lost a lot of weight, e.g., after bariatric surgery, should be reevaluated, ideally with a PSG to document the degree of improvement.

The extent of improvement usually depends upon the severity of preexisting apnea and is variable. Depending upon the results of the PSG after weight loss, they may require a lower CPAP level and occasionally require no CPAP at all.

87. My patient has undergone UPPP for OSA. Should he/she be reevaluated?

Ideally, patients should undergo a repeat PSG about 3 months after UPPP to document the severity of OSA for comparison with the preoperative situation. This is particularly important if the apnea was moderate to severe and surgery was performed because CPAP could not be used—in such cases, the apnea is usually not fully corrected and additional treatment may be required.

88. Which patients with sleep apnea should be reported to the authorities governing driving licensure?

This is a controversial issue. There is no "right answer", and the following statements may not meet with universal agreement.

Reporting of patients should be in accordance with local legislation, but such legislation is often open to interpretation. Although some may favour mandatory reporting of every patient with sleep apnea, it is the author's considered opinion that such a policy is neither necessary nor beneficial.

The decision to report should be based not simply on whether or not sleep apnea is present but whether or not there is a significant risk to the patient and others on the road due to sleepiness. The decision should take into account not only the severity of apnea but also the severity of symptoms, previous history of motor vehicle accidents, occupation, and response to treatment. There is some evidence that mandatory reporting of all patients with sleep apnea may reduce the chances of them seeking medical attention.

Patients who are to be reported should be made aware of this fact in advance. In the author's experience, reporting does not automatically mean that the driver's license is revoked. At least in Ontario, Canada, patients are given a few weeks time by the Ministry of Transportation, during which appropriate treatment can be instituted. Of course, local policies and regulations may vary. Patients who do lose their driving privileges should be given every opportunity to reclaim them by complying with treatment and improving their somnolence.

BIBLIOGRAPHY

- Stevens DR. Sleep medicine secrets. Hanley & Belfus Inc; 2004.

- Avidan AY, Zee PH. Handbook of sleep medicine. Lippincott Williams & Wilkins; 2006.

- Chokroverty S. Clinical companion to sleep disorders medicine, 2nd ed. Butterworth-Heinemann; 2000.

- Pagel JS, Pandi-Perumal SR, editors. Primary care sleep medicine. Humana Press Inc; 2007.

- Fleetham J, Ayas N, Bradley D, Ferguson K, Fitzpatrick M, George C, et al. Canadian Thoracic Society guidelines: diagnosis and treatment of sleep disordered breathing in adults. Can Resp J 2006;13(7):387-92.

- Kryger MH, Roth T, Dement WC. Principles and practice of sleep medicine, 4th ed. WB Saunders Co; 2005.

- Mazzagatti FA, Lebowitz LC, Schugler NW. Respiratory care pearls. Hanley & Belfus Inc; 1997.

- Abrams B. The perils of sleep apnea—an undiagnosed epidemic—a layman's perspective. iUniverse; 2007.

- Pascualy R. Snoring and sleep apnea—sleep well, feel better. 4th ed. Demos Medical Publishing; 2008.

INDEX

www.ingramcontent.com/pod-product-compliance
Lightning Source LLC
Chambersburg PA
CBHW031329290526
45784CB00014B/2448